The Consequences of Maternal Morbidity and Maternal Mortality

REPORT OF A WORKSHOP

Committee on Population

Holly E. Reed, Marjorie A. Koblinsky, and W. Henry Mosley, editors

Commission on Behavioral and Social Sciences and Education

National Research Council

NATIONAL ACADEMY PRESS
Washington, DC

NATIONAL ACADEMY PRESS • 2101 Constitution Ave., NW • Washington, DC 20418

NOTICE: The project that is the subject of this report was approved by the Governing Board of the National Research Council, whose members are drawn from the councils of the National Academy of Sciences, the National Academy of Engineering, and the Institute of Medicine. The members of the committee responsible for the report were chosen for their special competences and with regard for appropriate balance.

This project was funded by the William and Flora Hewlett Foundation, the Andrew W. Mellon Foundation, and the United States Agency for International Development. Any opinions, findings, conclusions, or recommendations expressed in this publication are those of the authors and do not necessarily reflect the views of the organizations that provided support for the project.

International Standard Book Number 0-309-06943-2

Suggested citation: National Research Council (2000) *The Consequences of Maternal Morbidity and Maternal Mortality: Report of a Workshop.* Committee on Population. Holly E. Reed, Marjorie A. Koblinsky, and W. Henry Mosley, editors. Commission on Behavioral and Social Sciences and Education. Washington, DC: National Academy Press.

Additional copies of this report are available from
National Academy Press
2101 Constitution Avenue, NW
Washington, DC 20418

Call 800-624-6242 or 202-334-3313 (in the Washington Metropolitan Area).
This report is also available on line at http://www.nap.edu

Printed in the United States of America

Copyright 2000 by the National Academy of Sciences. All rights reserved.

THE NATIONAL ACADEMIES

National Academy of Sciences
National Academy of Engineering
Institute of Medicine
National Research Council

The **National Academy of Sciences** is a private, nonprofit, self-perpetuating society of distinguished scholars engaged in scientific and engineering research, dedicated to the furtherance of science and technology and to their use for the general welfare. Upon the authority of the charter granted to it by the Congress in 1863, the Academy has a mandate that requires it to advise the federal government on scientific and technical matters. Dr. Bruce M. Alberts is president of the National Academy of Sciences.

The **National Academy of Engineering** was established in 1964, under the charter of the National Academy of Sciences, as a parallel organization of outstanding engineers. It is autonomous in its administration and in the selection of its members, sharing with the National Academy of Sciences the responsibility for advising the federal government. The National Academy of Engineering also sponsors engineering programs aimed at meeting national needs, encourages education and research, and recognizes the superior achievements of engineers. Dr. William A. Wulf is president of the National Academy of Engineering.

The **Institute of Medicine** was established in 1970 by the National Academy of Sciences to secure the services of eminent members of appropriate professions in the examination of policy matters pertaining to the health of the public. The Institute acts under the responsibility given to the National Academy of Sciences by its congressional charter to be an adviser to the federal government and, upon its own initiative, to identify issues of medical care, research, and education. Dr. Kenneth I. Shine is president of the Institute of Medicine.

The **National Research Council** was organized by the National Academy of Sciences in 1916 to associate the broad community of science and technology with the Academy's purposes of furthering knowledge and advising the federal government. Functioning in accordance with general policies determined by the Academy, the Council has become the principal operating agency of both the National Academy of Sciences and the National Academy of Engineering in providing services to the government, the public, and the scientific and engineering communities. The Council is administered jointly by both Academies and the Institute of Medicine. Dr. Bruce M. Alberts and Dr. William A. Wulf are chairman and vice chairman, respectively, of the National Research Council.

COMMITTEE ON POPULATION
1998

JANE MENKEN (*Chair*), Institute of Behavioral Sciences, University of Colorado, Boulder
CAROLINE H. BLEDSOE, Department of Anthropology, Northwestern University
JOHN BONGAARTS, Population Council, New York City
DAVID A. LAM, Population Studies Center, University of Michigan, Ann Arbor
LINDA G. MARTIN, RAND, Santa Monica, California
MARK R. MONTGOMERY, Population Council, New York City, and Department of Economics, State University of New York, Stony Brook
W. HENRY MOSLEY, Department of Population and Family Health Sciences, Johns Hopkins University
ALBERTO PALLONI, Center for Demography and Ecology, University of Wisconsin, Madison
JAMES P. SMITH, RAND, Santa Monica, California
BETH J. SOLDO, Department of Demography, Georgetown University
LINDA J. WAITE, Population Research Center, University of Chicago

BARNEY COHEN, *Director*
HOLLY REED, *Research Associate*
ELIZABETH WALLACE, *Project Assistant*

WORKSHOP ON THE CONSEQUENCES OF PREGNANCY, MATERNAL MORBIDITY, AND MORTALITY FOR WOMEN, THEIR FAMILIES, AND SOCIETY

Presenters

MARTHA AINSWORTH, World Bank, Washington, DC
ALAKA M. BASU, Division of Nutritional Sciences, Cornell University
JACQUELYN C. CAMPBELL, School of Nursing, Johns Hopkins University
WILLARD CATES, JR., Family Health International, Research Triangle Park, North Carolina
JULIA DAYTON, Department of Epidemiology and Public Health, Yale University
SONALDE DESAI, Department of Sociology, University of Maryland, College Park
STAN D'SOUZA, International Population Concerns, Brussels, Belgium
RONALD H. GRAY, School of Hygiene and Public Health, Johns Hopkins University
MARJORIE A. KOBLINSKY, MotherCare/John Snow, Inc., Arlington, Virginia
LISA M. LEE, Division of HIV/AIDS Prevention, Centers for Disease Control and Prevention, Atlanta, Georgia
REYNALDO MARTORELL, Department of International Health, Emory University
JANE MENKEN, Institute of Behavioral Sciences, University of Colorado, Boulder
KATHLEEN MERCHANT, Community Well-Being International, Henderson, Nevada
W. HENRY MOSLEY, Department of Population and Family Health Sciences, Johns Hopkins University
MEAD OVER, World Bank, Washington, DC
JOY RIGGS-PERLA, Center for Population, Health, and Nutrition, U.S. Agency for International Development
CARINE RONSMANS, Maternal and Child Epidemiology Unit, London School of Hygiene and Tropical Medicine, London
SHEA RUTSTEIN, Macro International, Calverton, Maryland
JASON B. SMITH, Family Health International, Research Triangle Park, North Carolina
MICHAEL A. STRONG, U.S. Agency for International Development, Nairobi, Kenya
ANNE TINKER, World Bank, Washington, DC
L. LEWIS WALL, Louisiana State University Medical Center, New Orleans, and School of Public Health, Tulane University
KEITH P. WEST, JR., School of Hygiene and Public Health, Johns Hopkins University

Other Participants

CARLA ABOUZAHR, World Health Organization, Geneva, Switzerland
JENNIFER ADAMS, Center for Population, Health, and Nutrition, U.S. Agency for International Development
FRANK ANDERSON, Bureau for Humanitarian Response, U.S. Agency for International Development
PATRICIA BAILEY, Family Health International, Research Triangle Park, North Carolina
ALFRED BARTLETT, Center for Population, Health, and Nutrition, U.S. Agency for International Development
INGVILD BELLE, Inter-American Development Bank, Washington, DC
CYNTHIA BERG, Centers for Disease Control and Prevention, U.S. Department of Health and Human Services, Atlanta, Georgia
CAROLINE H. BLEDSOE, Department of Anthropology, Northwestern University
ANNETTE BONGIOVANNI, Bureau for Latin America and the Caribbean, U.S. Agency for International Development
SANDRA DECASTRO BUFFINGTON, Center for Population, Health, and Nutrition, U.S. Agency for International Development
LATASHA COLE, Global Health Council, Washington, DC
COLLEEN CONROY, MotherCare/John Snow, Inc., Arlington, Virginia
COLLETTE CURRAN, Population Reference Bureau, Washington, DC
NILS DAULAIRE, Global Health Council, Washington, DC
PATRICIA DAVID, Population Reference Bureau, Washington, DC
FRANCE DONNAY, UNICEF, New York, New York
LESLIE ELDER, MotherCare/John Snow, Inc., Arlington, Virginia
PHYLLIS GESTRIN, Bureau for Africa, U.S. Agency for International Development
MOLLY GINGERICH, Center for Population, Health, and Nutrition, U.S. Agency for International Development
JOHN HAAGA, Population Reference Bureau, Washington, DC
SANDRA HUFFMAN, Academy for Educational Development, Washington, DC
ZAHID HUQUE, MotherCare/John Snow, Inc., Arlington, Virginia
EDNA JONAS, Consultant, Silver Spring, Maryland
KATHERINE JONES, Bureau for Humanitarian Response, U.S. Agency for International Development
MICHAEL KOENIG, School of Hygiene and Public Health, Johns Hopkins University
KATHERINE KRASOVEC, Abt Associates, Inc., Bethesda, Maryland
MIRIAM LABBOK, Center for Population, Health, and Nutrition, U.S. Agency for International Development

JEANNE McDERMOTT, MotherCare/John Snow, Inc., Arlington, Virginia
THOMAS MERRICK, World Bank, Washington, DC
MAUREEN NORTON, Center for Population, Health, and Nutrition, U.S. Agency for International Development
SHIRLIE PINKHAM, Bureau for Population, Refugees, and Migration, U.S. Department of State
MIRIAM SCHNEIDMAN, World Bank, Washington, DC
ELISABETH SOMMERFELT, JHPIEGO Corporation, Baltimore, Maryland
MARY ELLEN STANTON, Center for Population, Health, and Nutrition, U.S. Agency for International Development
ANN STARRS, Family Care International, New York, New York
PATRICIA STEPHENSON, Center for Population, Health, and Nutrition, U.S. Agency for International Development
KRISTA STEWART, Center for Population, Health, and Nutrition, U.S. Agency for International Development
REMA VENU, UNICEF, New York, New York
VIRGINIA VITZTHUM, Center for Population, Health, and Nutrition, U.S. Agency for International Development
BEVERLY WINIKOFF, Population Council, New York

FAITH MITCHELL, *Director*, Division on Social and Economic Studies
BARNEY COHEN, *Director*, Committee on Population
HOLLY E. REED, *Research Associate*, Committee on Population
ELIZABETH WALLACE, *Project Assistant*, Committee on Population

Contents

Preface	xi
Introduction	1
Framing the Subject: What Is Known About Maternal Morbidity and Mortality	3
Evidence on the Consequences of Maternal Mortality	5
Evidence on the Consequences of Maternal Morbidity	11
Opportunities for Further Research	17
References	19
Appendix A: Definitions	23
Appendix B: Workshop Agenda	26

Preface

The National Research Council (NRC) established the Committee on Population in 1983 to bring the knowledge and methods of the population sciences to bear on major issues of science and public policy. The committee's work includes both basic studies of fertility, health and mortality, and migration, and applied studies aimed at improving programs for the public health and welfare in the United States and developing countries. The committee also fosters communication among researchers in different disciplines and countries and policy makers in government and international agencies.

In 1997 the committee published *Reproductive Health in Developing Countries: Expanding Dimensions, Building Solutions*, a report that recommended actions to improve reproductive health for women around the world. As a follow-on activity, the committee proposed an investigation into the social and economic consequences of maternal morbidity and mortality. With funding from the William and Flora Hewlett Foundation, the Andrew W. Mellon Foundation, and the U.S. Agency for International Development, the committee organized a workshop on this topic in Washington, DC, on October 19-20, 1998.

A Committee on Population workshop is intended to be a stimulating forum for leading scientists and policy makers from a variety of different disciplines to discuss what is known about a particular scientific topic. The Workshop on the Consequences of Pregnancy, Maternal Morbidity, and Mortality for Women, Their Families, and Society brought together researchers from the fields of anthropology, demography, economics, medicine, public health, and sociology and policy makers from government agencies, nongovernmental, and international organizations. The goal of the workshop was to assess the existing scientific knowledge about the consequences of maternal morbidity and mortality and to discuss key findings from recent research. Although the existing research on this topic is scarce, presenters drew on similar literature on the consequences of adult disease and death, especially the growing literature on the socioeconomic consequences of AIDS, to look at potential consequences from maternal disability and death.

Given the limitations of both time and scope that are inherent to a workshop, some other important topics could not be addressed. These included: the consequences of several types of morbidities, such as prolapse, eclampsia, ectopic pregnancy, and complications from unsafe abortion; the psychosocial affects of maternal morbidity and mortality; the fiscal costs of reproductive disability and death; and the changes in social structure that may result from maternal morbidity and mortality. The fact that they were not discussed does not indicate that they are not important topics deserving of future consideration.

This report summarizes the presentations and discussion at the workshop. Although some references are provided, it is by no means a comprehensive review of the subject. It is hoped that this report will encourage further investigation into the consequences of maternal morbidity and mortality.

I am grateful to my fellow committee members, Caroline Bledsoe, John Bongaarts, and Henry Mosley, who served with me on the subcommittee that organized the workshop. In addition, the committee was extremely fortunate in being able to enlist the services of Marge Koblinsky, one of the leading experts in this field. She collaborated with the committee members, provided valuable advice and direction during the planning stages of the meeting, and cochaired the meeting with Henry Mosley. Keith West, from the Johns Hopkins University and Leslie Elder, from John Snow, Inc. both helped to review the section on nutrition in this report.

The staff at the National Research Council managed the workshop from start to finish and made it all possible. Holly Reed, research associate, helped develop the framework for the workshop, coordinated the contributions of the participants, and worked with Marge Koblinsky and Henry Mosley to produce this report. Elizabeth Wallace, project assistant, assisted with logistical and travel arrangements for the workshop. Eugenia Grohman, associate director for reports for the Commission on Behavioral and Social Sciences and Education, skillfully edited the manuscript and guided it through the review process. The work was carried out under the general direction of Barney Cohen.

This report has been reviewed in draft form by individuals chosen for their diverse perspectives and technical expertise, in accordance with procedures approved by the NRC's Report Review Committee. The purpose of this independent review is to provide candid and critical comments that will assist the institution in making the published report as sound as possible and to ensure that the report meets institutional standards for objectivity, evidence, and responsiveness

PREFACE   xiii

to the study charge. The review comments and draft manuscript remain confidential to protect the integrity of the deliberative process.

We wish to thank the following individuals for their participation in the review of this report: Oona Campbell, Maternal and Child Epidemiology Unit, London School of Hygiene and Tropical Medicine; David A. Lam, Population Studies Center, University of Michigan, Ann Arbor; Deborah Maine, School of Public Health, Columbia University; T. Paul Schultz, Department of Economics, Yale University; and John Strauss, Department of Economics, Michigan State University.

Although the individuals listed above have provided constructive comments and suggestions, it must be emphasized that responsibility for the final content of this report rests entirely with the authoring committee and the institution.

The work of the committee and the NRC, however, could not be done without the valuable contributions of experts who present their research and viewpoints in workshops like the one on which this report is based. (See Appendix B for the workshop agenda.) We are most grateful to these dedicated workshop participants, whose ideas and discussions are summarized here. We hope that this publication helps ensure that their work will continue to contribute to research and policy on reproductive and maternal morbidity and maternal mortality and their consequences.

Jane Menken, *Chair*
Committee on Population

The Consequences of Maternal Morbidity and Maternal Mortality

INTRODUCTION

Current best estimates indicate that more than 54 million women suffer from diseases or complications during pregnancy and childbirth and more than one-half million women die of causes related to pregnancy and childbirth each year (World Health Organization, 1993; World Health Organization and United Nations Children's Fund, 1996). To a greater or lesser extent, the risk of death from complications arising during pregnancy affects women in every country in the world.

In 1987 the global "Safe Motherhood Initiative" was launched by a group of international agencies at an international conference in Nairobi, Kenya, with the ambitious goal of reducing maternal mortality by half by the year 2000. The initiative has contributed much to knowledge of the causes of maternal morbidity and mortality and has been instrumental in advocating for improved access to health care for women, but the goal of halving the number of maternal deaths globally has yet to be achieved. In fact, expert opinion puts the annual number of deaths globally due to complications during pregnancy higher than it was 10 years ago.

Table 1 shows the best available estimates of maternal mortality ratios, total maternal deaths, and lifetime risk of maternal death in the developing world in 1983 and 1990. The global maternal mortality ratio in 1983 was estimated to be 390 maternal deaths per 100,000 live births; in 1990, it was estimated to be 430. The approximate lifetime risk of maternal death was estimated at 1 in 58 in 1983 and 1 in 60 in 1990. Similarly, the total number of maternal deaths was estimated at about 500,000 per year in 1983 and about 585,000 per year in 1990; the regions

TABLE 1 Maternal Mortality Ratio, Number of Maternal Deaths, and Lifetime Risk of Maternal Death, World and Developing Regions, 1983 and 1990

U.N. Region	Maternal Mortality Ratio[a]		Maternal Deaths		Lifetime Risk of Maternal Death, 1 in:	
	1983	1990	1983	1990	1983	1990
World	390	430	500,000	585,000	58	60
More developed regions	30	27	6,000	4,000	N/A	1,800
Less developed regions	450	480	494,000	582,000	N/A	48
Africa	640	870	150,000	235,000	21	16
Northern Africa	500	340	24,000	16,000	28	55
Western Africa	700	1,020	54,000	87,000	19	12
Eastern Africa	660	1,060	46,000	97,000	19	12
Middle Africa	690	950	18,000	31,000	20	14
Southern Africa	570	260	8,000	3,600	29	75
Asia	420	390	308,000	323,000	54	65
Western Asia	340	320	14,000	16,000	34	55
Southern Asia	650	560	230,000	227,000	26	35
Southeastern Asia	420	440	52,000	56,000	44	55
East Asia	55	95	12,000	24,000	722	410
Latin America and the Caribbean	270	190	34,000	23,000	N/A	130
Middle America	240	140	9,000	4,700	N/A	170
Caribbean	220	400	2,000	3,200	N/A	75
Tropical South America	310	200	22,000	15,000	N/A	140
Temperate South America	110	200	1,000	15,000	N/A	140
Oceania	N/A	680	2,000	1,400	N/A	26

[a]Maternal deaths per 100,000 live births.
SOURCE: Data for 1983 from AbouZahr and Royston (1991: Table 2.1); data for 1990 from World Health Organization and United Nations Children's Fund (1996: Table 1). Reprinted with permission.

with the largest numbers of maternal deaths are Africa and Asia. At first glance, it appears that maternal mortality increased between 1983 and 1990, but in reality differences between the two estimates is almost certainly a reflection of the alternative strategies used for estimation (World Health Organization and United Nations Children's Fund, 1996). Despite this potential confusion in interpreting the data, it seems clear that maternal mortality ratios are not declining at a rate that would achieve the 1987 goal for the year 2000.

Continued high levels of maternal morbidity and mortality have consequences that affect women, their children, their families, and even their communities. In an attempt to learn more about the potential consequences of maternal morbidity and mortality, the Committee on Population convened the Workshop on the Consequences of Pregnancy, Maternal Morbidity, and Mortality for Women, Their Families, and Society at the National Academies in Washington, D.C. The workshop was intended to serve as a first step towards a better understanding of how reproductive illness, disability, and death, especially during pregnancy and childbirth, affect women, their children and families, and their communities. The purpose of the workshop was not to reach consensus about such consequences, but rather to explore some of the potential links between maternal morbidity, maternal mortality, and their consequences.

Research on the outcomes resulting from reproductive morbidity or maternal morbidity or mortality is still in its infancy. To a large extent, the workshop presentations highlighted the scarcity of good research in this area. Workshop participants included policy makers, reproductive health program managers, representatives of international organizations, and researchers from demography, medicine, sociology, economics, public health, and population policy. Twelve presentations covered a range of topics related to maternal morbidity and mortality. These topics are by no means a comprehensive review of the field. But they reflect the kind of research that is actively taking place in this area. Taken collectively, the presentations at the workshop shed some new light on the effects of maternal morbidity and mortality on the lives of women, children, and families.

FRAMING THE SUBJECT: WHAT IS KNOWN ABOUT MATERNAL MORBIDITY AND MORTALITY?

Maternal morbidity and mortality are usually defined as morbidities or mortality that occur during pregnancy or childbirth or within 42 days after giving birth. (See Appendix A for detailed definitions.) Reproductive morbidity includes maternal (or obstetric) morbidity, gynecologic morbidity, and contraceptive morbidity. Maternal morbidity, which is a part of reproductive morbidity, is generally defined as any illness or injury caused by, aggravated by, or associated with pregnancy or childbirth. Maternal mortality, defined as death during pregnancy or childbirth, or within 42 days after giving birth, can include direct causes (acute problems such as obstetric complications) and indirect causes (problems that are not necessarily caused by the pregnancy, but rather aggravated by the pregnant state, such as anemia or malaria). Sexually transmitted diseases, including HIV/AIDS, are gynecologic morbidities. These definitions are clearly quite broad. Yet by beginning with a wide scope, it may be easier to capture all of the possible consequences that reproductive morbidity and maternal morbidity could have.

In developing countries, pregnancy and childbirth-related complications are the leading cause of disability and one of the leading causes of death among

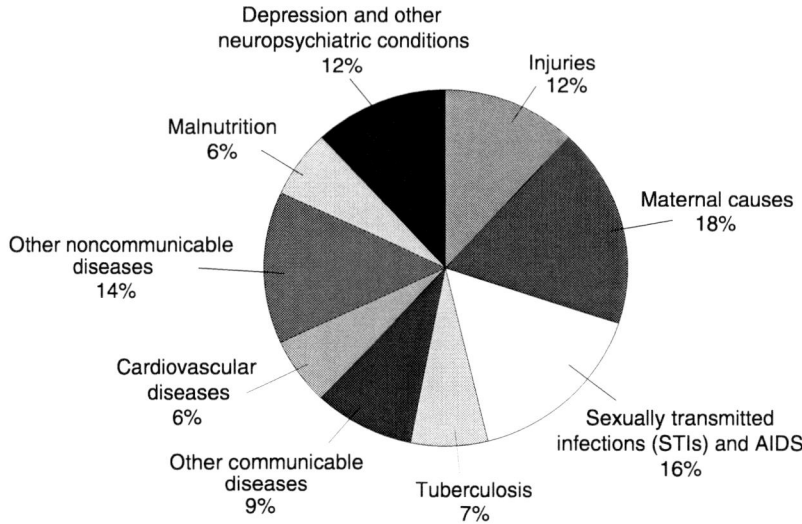

FIGURE 1 Burden of disease in females aged 15-44 in developing countries. SOURCE: World Bank (1993: Figure 2.3). Reprinted with permission.

women aged 15-44. The World Development Report estimated that 18 percent of the burden of disease for these women is due to maternal causes (see Figure 1). An additional 16 percent of the burden of disease is due to AIDS and other sexually transmitted infections, which can often lead to or exacerbate problems in pregnancy and childbirth (World Bank, 1993). The most frequent causes of maternal mortality are severe bleeding, responsible for 25 percent of the deaths; indirect causes, such as complications related to anemia, malaria, and heart disease, responsible for another 20 percent of maternal mortality globally; and infection or sepsis, responsible for 15 percent of the deaths (see Figure 2). These numbers, which were published by the World Health Organization, are only best guesses, because there are no reliable population-based statistics on the causes of maternal mortality in most parts of the world, but they provide a general idea of the scope of the problem.

When a woman dies or becomes ill or injured either during or shortly after giving birth, the consequences have the potential to affect no only the woman herself, but her family and her community in a variety of ways; see Table 2. Morbidity and mortality can have health effects and psychological costs for women, children, and other family or household members. In addition, children's schooling, supervision, and care may be affected by their mother's morbidity or mortality. There are also potential family or household economic costs associ-

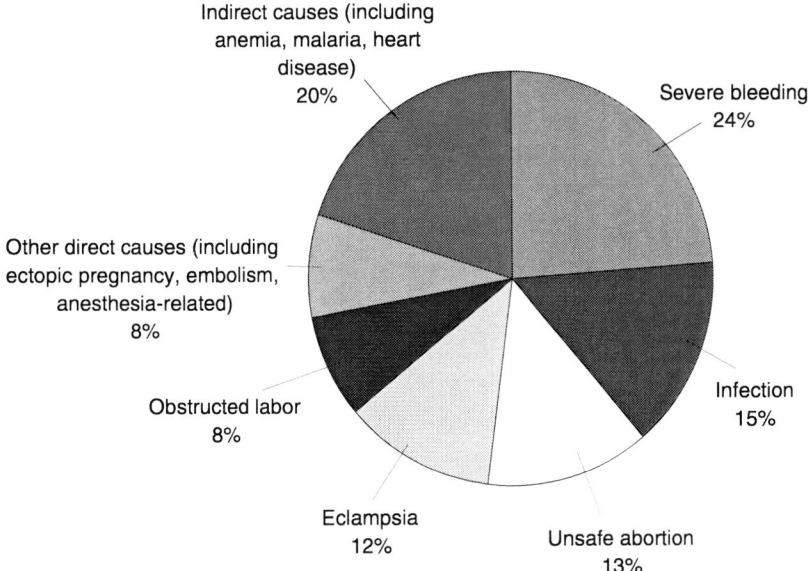

FIGURE 2 Causes of maternal death worldwide. SOURCE: World Health Organization (1997: Figure 1). Reprinted with permission.

ated with illness and death, including changes in labor allocation, productivity, consumption, investment, and direct costs, such as medical or funeral expenditures. Finally, community and even societal norms and behaviors may be affected by illness or death, especially if the sick or deceased woman is or was a prominent member of the community. As for all adult illness and death, the response from the household, community, and society determines whether a family, community, or society can cope with the consequences of maternal morbidity and mortality. The consequences may differ substantially depending on the roles of the family member who is sick or who dies.

EVIDENCE ON THE CONSEQUENCES OF MATERNAL MORTALITY

The potential social and economic consequences of maternal mortality seem obvious, but in fact they have not been demonstrated, partly due to measurement problems. Henry Mosley noted that the consequences of maternal mortality are extremely difficult to measure, because it is a relatively rare demographic event. For example, if the maternal mortality ratio is about 400 deaths per 100,000 live births, one would have to follow an average population of 500,000 annually for 5 years to observe 400 maternal deaths. This rarity makes it challenging to separate

TABLE 2 Potential Effects on Children, Families and Households, and Communities and Society Due to Maternal Morbidity and Maternal Mortality

Potential Effects	On Children	On Families and Households	On Communities and Society
Demographic	Death	Loss of deceased Dissolution or reconstitution of family/household	Loss of deceased Increased number of one-parent households Increased number of orphans
Economic	Increased labor force participation	Reduced productivity of ill adult Lost output of deceased adult Reallocation of land and labor Medical costs of treatment Dissaving Changes in consumption and investment Funeral costs, legal fees Transfers Changes in household management	Reduced productivity of ill adult Lost output of deceased adult Reallocation of land and labor Dissaving Changes in consumption and investment Transfers Economic burden of one-parent
Health	Illness Injury Malnutrition Poor hygiene	Reduced allocation of labor to health maintaining activities Poor health for surviving household members	Change in the allocation of labor to health maintaining activities
Psychological	Depression Other psychological problems	Depression Other psychological problems Grief of loved ones	Grief Loss of community cohesion
Social	Social isolation Reduced education Reduced parental supervision and care	Social isolation Changes in care for children, elderly, and disabled	Changes in responsibility for care of children, elderly, and disabled Loss of community/societal leaders Changes in women's rights, health policy, other public policy

maternal mortality from female deaths in general, so maternal mortality studies generally have a special surveillance system set up in a large population (Chen et al., 1983; Egypt Ministry of Health, 1994).

Because of these measurement difficulties, the workshop presentations often examined the impact of a mother's death from any cause on her children, family, and household. Studies of adult mortality in general, including that due to AIDS, were presented when data on the consequences of maternal mortality in particular were unavailable. It is also important to note that households that experience an adult death may have been economically and socially disadvantaged before the death occurred. Selection bias, therefore, has the potential to affect the results of this research. The studies that were discussed during the workshop are detailed below, but again it must be recognized that they do not cover the entire spectrum of potential consequences.

Direct Evidence: Consequences for Children

The workshop included presentations of several studies on the effects that maternal mortality has on children's health and well-being. The key findings from these studies are summarized below. As previously noted, this summary is not a comprehensive review of the research on this issue, but it highlights several consequences of maternal mortality for children that were presented at the workshop, including increased mortality risk, decreased nutrition, and decreased schooling.

Increased Mortality Risk for Children

Strong described a study in Matlab, Bangladesh, between 1983 and 1987 (Strong, 1998). Children 0 to 9 years of age whose households experienced an adult death from any cause in their household were monitored for 2 years. The results of the logistic regression analysis showed that children whose mothers died were much more likely to die than those whose fathers died, and both groups had higher mortality than children whose households did not experience an adult death. Most deaths were among children under 1 year old. After the first month of life, female children were much more likely than male children to die.

Decreased Nutrition and Schooling for Children

There are few available data on the effects of maternal deaths on children's overall welfare, but some research has looked at the effects of parental death on the nutritional status and schooling of children. Martha Ainsworth described her longitudinal study with Innocent Semali in the Kagera region of Tanzania, on the effects of parental death on children's nutritional status (Ainsworth and Semali, 1998). This area has high rates of HIV infection and AIDS, and anthropometric data show very high levels of stunting (low height for age) among children under 5 years of age. The results from random-effects and fixed-effects regression models showed that children who lost their mothers were much more likely to be stunted than children who lost their fathers or than children with both parents living. The children who were most affected were children who lost their mothers and whose mothers had no education. The link to education may be because mother's education is a proxy for the socioeconomic status of the household (Ainsworth and Semali, 1998).

Ainsworth and Semali (1998) also studied the effect of the deaths of prime-aged adults in a household (not necessarily parents) on the stunting of children under age 5. In the Kagera region of Tanzania, adult deaths are more likely to occur in households with relatively higher socioeconomic status. Following an adult death in the household, stunting in children increased to levels found in households that did not suffer an adult death and who are generally less wealthy.

Ainsworth also discussed the effects that parental deaths had on children's schooling in the Kagera region. Children who had lost their mothers or fathers or both had somewhat lower school enrollment rates overall. However, children who had lost a parent in the poorest households had the lowest enrollment rates; those in relatively better off households had enrollment rates similar to children with both parents living. The most striking result of the study was that the death of a prime-aged female adult—whether or not she was a parent—resulted in delayed school enrollment of both boys and girls aged 7-11 and early dropouts among children aged 15-19. The death of a prime-aged male did not have any effect on enrollment. This finding suggests that teenage children are important substitutes for women's time in home production activities.

Indirect Evidence:
Consequences of Parental Mortality for Families and Society

Although a woman's children may shoulder the greatest burden of their mother's death, the entire family is likely to suffer. However, the overall consequences for society from maternal mortality alone are likely to be modest for two reasons: maternal mortality is a relatively infrequent cause of adult death in high mortality settings, and women's measurable productive contributions in developing countries are often less relevant than the noneconomic benefits that she brings to her family. The following section summarizes the potential consequences for families and society that were presented at the workshop. Obviously there are many topics that warrant further exploration.

Studies of Adult Mortality and Poverty

Stan D'Souza presented data from two bivariate studies of the social and economic consequences of parental death in Kinshasa, Zaire (now the Democratic Republic of Congo), and Kigali, Rwanda. In Kinshasa, coping strategies were examined for households where the household head died, usually a man. D'Souza found that most of the poorest households were headed by widows, but the effect was mitigated somewhat if the widow had a small business or if the family structure was matrilineal, allowing her more access to family resources. The income provided by children's labor appeared to be important for widows' survival, while education was often postponed for those children who lost a parent. Sometimes children worked in the informal sector or as prostitutes, trying to make enough money to buy food for themselves or to help support their families (D'Souza, 1994).

The Kigali data were collected in 1996, immediately before approximately 1,000,000 refugees returned to Rwanda following the massive genocide and its aftermath of revenge killings that resulted in an estimated 800,000 to 1,000,000 dead or missing people. Nearly every family had lost at least one male family member. The percentage of women in the 20-44 and 45-64 age groups was more than 57 percent. Consequently, much of the sample comprised households that contained widows and their children: 68 percent of female heads of households were widows. Children were often separated from their families and suffered severe psychological trauma due to the violence they had witnessed (D'Souza et al., 1998).

The Kigali and Kinshasa studies, along with illustrations from the ongoing longitudinal database in Matlab, Bangladesh, emphasized the two-way linkages between a death in a family and poverty. When an adult family member dies, particularly the breadwinner of the household, families may face economic insecurity or poverty. A poor family is economically vulnerable and susceptible to malnutrition, infectious diseases, and lack of education. These circumstances in turn continue the cycle of death and poverty (D'Souza, 1994).

Studies of Adult Mortality and Household Consumption

The death of an adult may affect the level of household consumption, mostly because of smaller household size and reduced resources for purchasing food and other necessary items. Over and Dayton found a pattern of death and poverty in the Kagera region of Tanzania, due to the AIDS epidemic there (World Bank, 1997). Using logistic regression models, they examined household consumption following the death of an adult in comparison with consumption in households that did not experience an adult death. Obviously, the households in which adults had died usually had large expenditures for medical and funeral expenses. Other nonfood expenditures were lower: households often increased their home food production (e.g., gardening) to compensate for reduced food expenditures. Thus, controlling for other factors, there did not appear to be a clear difference in the overall level of food consumption per capita in households with and without an adult death, indicating that home food production probably made up for any reduction in purchased food.

Although death alone did not appear to affect consumption patterns in Tanzania, in combination with other factors it did have an effect. The most important indicator of reduced consumption was the level of household assets. In nonpoor households, there was actually an increase in consumption expenditures after a death (perhaps due to funeral and burial expenses), while in the poorest 50 percent of households, food expenditures dropped by almost one-third. This was somewhat compensated for by increasing home food production, but food consumption also dropped by about 15 percent in the poorest households. According to Over, it appeared that the death of an adult woman had the biggest effect on household consumption in the poorest households, at least for the year following the death.

Over noted that another important aspect of the relationship between death in the household and consumption is assistance from outside sources. Households that experienced a death received only slightly higher public transfers, but private transfers were much greater following a death in this African setting. Family assistance is more important than government aid in helping families to cope with the loss of a family member. The households that did receive public transfers were the poorest households, so some targeted assistance may be occurring.

In sum, according to Over, the link between death in the household and poverty is very complex in the Kagera region. Households have a variety of techniques to cope with adult death, such as increased home food production. The poorest households suffer the most in terms of reduced consumption, so assistance programs that are targeted towards these households have the potential to be the most effective.

Studies of Adult Mortality and Household Management

In addition to direct economic effects, the death of an adult can affect how a household is managed, especially if the deceased was the primary household manager. Alaka Basu examined the potential effects of adult mortality on household management in a survey of households in New Delhi, India. India has a very poor social safety net and virtually no health insurance, so medical costs are borne almost entirely by families. Basu's explanatory study attempted to determine what the coping mechanisms are in Delhi for a family that loses an adult family member and how long the family could cope with a death without having to drastically change its life-style. It is important to remember that many urban dwellers in India live in nuclear families and often do not have the assistance of extended kin networks; hence, coping with an adult death may be more difficult for them than it would be for some rural dwellers.

The results indicated that nuclear families whose income came from the formal wage or salary sector were the worst off following an adult death in the household. Families living with extended kin who were self-employed were best able to cope with the loss. Work is often more flexible for the self-employed, which allows economic flexibility in dealing with the death of a family member. Households where women worked outside the home prior to the death were also better off, compared with more traditional households where women only worked in the home. Nevertheless, even the most flexible and nontraditional households eventually needed to rely on assistance from their extended families following an adult death in the household (Basu, 1998).

The largest economic effect of a death in the family appeared to occur when women died. It was often difficult for the household to survive, because men were unaccustomed to managing the household budget and affairs. Older children often had to drop out of school in order to work to help support the family; in other cases, they were sent to live with their grandparents (Basu, 1998).

Several participants noted that, in developing countries, it is the more "modern," middle-class families who are often hardest hit by a death in the household because they have weaker safety nets. "Traditional" family structures appear to be a better coping mechanism for dealing with adult death. The families in Basu's (1998) study had a hard time coping with the loss of a mother mainly because they had lost their "home economist," and a mother's skills are often difficult to replace.

EVIDENCE ON THE CONSEQUENCES OF MATERNAL MORBIDITY

The World Health Organization estimates that 42 percent of the approximately 129 million women who give birth annually (according to the United Nations) experience at least mild complications during pregnancy (United Nations, 1999; World Health Organization, 1993). Furthermore, an estimated 15 million women annually develop long-term disabilities due to pregnancy-related complications (World Health Organization, 1993). Despite the large numbers of women who are estimated to be affected by such morbidity, little is known about the interrelationships between different types of morbidities and their social and economic consequences. Many of these potentially adverse health consequences are difficult to measure, so the health effects of maternal morbidity are not well documented. There is even less knowledge about the psychological, social, and economic consequences.

Direct Evidence: Consequences for Women

Death is obviously the most serious consequence of maternal morbidity for women, yet maternal morbidity can lead to other severe consequences. Maternal morbidities can be acute, occurring during childbirth and immediately thereafter, or chronic, lasting for months or years. Many of these morbidities are conditions that may cause difficulty in pregnancy or aggravate existing morbidities, which can lead to more severe consequences for women. The workshop presentations highlighted some of the physical and mental consequences of maternal morbidity for women. As noted previously, the presentations did not cover every type of morbidity and possible adverse health and economic outcome, but instead focused on critical areas where current research is emerging. The workshop presentations made it clear that further research on the effects of various types of maternal morbidities is needed.

Consequences of Obstructed and Prolonged Labor

When a woman is unable to give birth vaginally due to malpresentation of the fetus, cephalopelvic disproportion, or other reasons, obstructed labor occurs. Most women in developed countries generally have the option of a cesarean section birth to avoid potential injury or death for themselves and the fetus. Yet throughout much of the developing world, women do not have any access to physicians, especially physicians trained to deal with obstructed labor. Obstructed labor can lead to uterine rupture, vaginal tears, the formation of an obstetric fistula,[1] and fetal asphyxia. The incontinence of urine (and sometimes feces) caused by a fistula can produce a foul odor and lead to feelings of shame or humiliation. Other injuries that can be caused by prolonged obstructed labor include renal failure, pelvic inflammatory disease, infertility, and neurological injuries, including a condition called foot drop caused by nerve damage to the lower spine (Arrowsmith et al., 1996).

Although surgical procedures can repair fistulas, many women in developing countries do not have access to this procedure. For example, obstetric fistulas occur throughout rural sub-Saharan Africa, where many women give birth with only the assistance of a traditional birth attendant. Yet there are only two prominent fistula hospitals in the whole sub-Saharan region, one in northern Nigeria and one in Addis Ababa, Ethiopia.

There are a number of adverse economic and social consequences associated with these conditions. Reporting on medical records obtained from the Addis Ababa Fistula Hospital and based on his own clinical experience, Lewis Wall noted that fistulas and other injuries associated with obstructed labor are not only extremely painful and uncomfortable, but the shame and social isolation they often cause can lead to depression, isolation, divorce, and even suicide. For example, women suffering from pelvic injuries and foot drop have difficulty completing such daily tasks as carrying water and firewood or caring for their children. Consequently, these women may be viewed as a burden to the family.

---

[1] An obstetric fistula is a hole between the vaginal wall and the bladder (vesico-vaginal fistula), the rectum, (recto-vaginal fistula), or both.

Women who are unable to have sexual intercourse or who are infertile due to fistula injuries are often shunned and abandoned by their husbands and families. Young women, often giving birth for the first time, seem to suffer fistulas more often than older women. As a consequence, the majority of vesico-vaginal fistula patients have no living children. In addition, the obviously unclean state of women with fistulas leads many African religious groups to prohibit their participation in forms of worship (Arrowsmith et al., 1996).

Workshop participants noted that there are important geographic variations in the prevalence of obstetric fistulas; specifically, they appear to be more common in sub-Saharan Africa than in other parts of the developing world (Cottingham and Royston, 1991). Although it is unclear why these differences exist, risk factors include young age at first birth, inadequate obstetric care, small body frames, and flat pelvises. Wall stated that several of these factors are common in African populations, including inadequate obstetric care, and young age at first birth. Yet many Asian populations, such as women in Bangladesh, do not exhibit high rates of fistula, despite apparent risk factors, such as small body frames and very poor access to obstetric care. Participants noted the relatively low average birthweight of Asian babies as a possible explanation. Another explanation explored by participants was the prevalence of the practice of female genital cutting in Africa, which can cause difficulties in labor and delivery. Wall, however, argued that female genital cutting has been overemphasized in connection with obstructed labor because the obstruction usually occurs higher up in the pelvic region. Instead, he emphasized the relatively low socioeconomic status of women in many African societies and the possibility that fistula patients may be more visible in areas with special treatment facilities, such as northern Nigeria and Addis Ababa. More research is needed in order to understand if there are geographic variations in the prevalence of obstetric fistula and if so, why these variations exist.

Without getting into the details of the cost-effectiveness of various potential interventions, participants discussed, in general terms, the question of how obstructed labor can be prevented. The first goal of primary prevention should be to increase women's age at first childbirth, to reduce the very risky pregnancies among very young women, although the association between age and risk of maternal mortality has not been proven (National Research Council, 1989). Second, programs should attempt to increase access to good quality, low-cost contraceptives, so that unwanted pregnancies or pregnancies with a known medical risk are avoided. Improved nutrition for girls and young women and the reduction of harmful practices, such as female genital cutting, may also reduce the chances of obstructed labor, although the links between these practices and maternal mortality are not established. Even with a reduction in risky pregnancies, secondary prevention will still be needed; increased access to essential obstetric care will be necessary to manage prolonged obstructed labor and its consequences (World Health Organization, 1994).

The Link Between HIV/AIDS and Other Sexually Transmitted Infections and Maternal Morbidity

HIV/AIDS and other sexually transmitted infections (STIs) are estimated to account for 16 percent of the burden of disease for females aged 15 to 44 in developing countries (Figure 1). These reproductive morbidities can affect both women's lives and the lives of their newborn children in a variety of ways, including reduced fertility for women. Ronald Gray and Lisa Lee discussed research on the effect of HIV/AIDS on fertility, using data from Rakai district, Uganda, and from the state of Maryland in the United States, respectively. Using bivariate and logistic regression analyses, the Rakai study examined pregnancy rates in relation to HIV and syphilis. Women who had neither infection had significantly higher pregnancy rates than women with early syphilis, HIV, or both (Gray et al., 1998). Gray hypothesized that a causal link between HIV and reduced fertility might be due to HIV itself or to a relationship between HIV and undiagnosed tubal infertility due to pelvic inflammatory disease (PID).

Lee described a similar study in Maryland, which confirmed those results. Using a linked database containing Medicaid enrollment and claims data, HIV/AIDS registry data, and vital statistics, the birth rates and pregnancy outcomes of women who were HIV-infected were compared with those who were not infected. HIV-positive women had reduced fertility in comparison with those who were not infected. The results also showed that the reduction in fertility in HIV-positive women becomes more pronounced with longer duration of HIV infection.

In addition to HIV/AIDS, there are a variety of other STIs that can affect women's health and fertility and the health and survival of newborns. Based on his many years of experience in this field, Ward Cates discussed the effects of such STIs as chlamydia and gonorrhea on PID and subsequent tubal infertility. Cates reported that it is difficult to establish direct links between STIs and tubal infertility. Most women who have tubal infertility have no documented past history of PID (Cates, 1995). Cates surmised that it is quite possible that some women were either misdiagnosed or never diagnosed and may not have even recognized any symptoms. However, past infection with chlamydia or gonorrhea is a strong risk factor for tubal infertility: it is estimated that almost 80 percent of tubal infertility in Africa is related to STIs (Cates, 1995).

New screening technologies are being developed for diseases like chlamydia, which is highly prevalent in many developing countries, especially among young women (Cates, 1995). Other infections, such as bacterial vaginosis and trichomonasis, are also highly prevalent in many developed and developing countries and have been linked to preterm births and the spread of AIDS. Gray stated that a dose of 2 grams of metronidazole and 1 gram of Azithromycin given to pregnant women was associated with improvement in birthweight and reduction in neonatal eye infection, probably as a consequence of reductions in bacterial vaginosis, gonorrhea, and chlamydia. These drugs are not harmful to pregnant women or to fetuses. Jane Menken recommended that a clinical trial study be undertaken to replicate these findings. Other suggested next steps included acquiring more information on levels of knowledge of women about STIs and their effects on themselves and their future children and learning more about cost-effective prevention and treatment for all types of STIs.

The Link Between Malnutrition and Maternal and Child Morbidity and Mortality

Women's malnutrition can have severe consequences, including reproductive and maternal morbidities and even death. For example, if a woman develops severe anemia (most commonly caused by iron deficiency), she can have a higher risk of dying during childbirth (Llewellyn-Jones, 1965; Harrison et al., 1985). Chronic undernutrition and specific micronutrient deficiencies are likely to make women less resistant to infections, a particularly frequent cause of morbidity, and there is some evidence that other conditions, such as eclampsia, may be exacerbated by specific nutrient deficiencies.

Intrauterine and early postnatal malnutrition can lead to growth failure in early life due to compromised oxygen delivery and impaired cardiovascular functioning. These are important determinants of short stature in women. Short maternal stature (stunting), in turn, is a known risk factor for obstructed labor and poor reproductive health outcomes. Therefore, preventing intrauterine and early childhood malnutrition may be important for reducing the risk of cephalopelvic disproportion and, perhaps, maternal mortality.

Specific micronutrient deficiencies are associated with negative effects on the health and survival of pregnant and lactating women and their offspring. For example, gestational zinc deficiency, which is likely to be widespread in many developing countries, may alter neurobehavioral development of the fetus (Merialdi et al., 1999), and it may predispose infants to early morbidity risk as it has been shown to do in preschool-aged children (Black, 1998).

Maternal iodine deficiency can cause a range of pathological conditions, including: abortions, stillbirths, brain damage, irreversible mental retardation, fetal growth retardation, and, cretinism. Mild neonatal iodine deficiency may increase risk of infant mortality (Cobra et al., 1997).

Moderate to severe anemia in pregnancy has been associated with low birthweight (Murphy et al., 1986) and prematurity (Zhou et al., 1998); in one recent trial, iron supplementation during pregnancy improved early infant survival (Preziosi et al., 1997; Christian et al., 1998a). The maternal health risks associated with widespread mild anemia have not yet been established, but at moderate levels of anemia, work capacity is impaired due to a combination of reduced oxygen-carrying capacity and the negative effect of iron deficiency on muscle function (Yip, 1994).

Recent evidence links vitamin A deficiency to multiple health risks for pregnant women. For example, maternal night blindness, due to vitamin A deficiency, occurs in 10 to 20 percent of pregnant women in malnourished, South Asian populations (Katz et al., 1995). Night blindness is associated with increased risks of wasting, anemia, infectious disease, and a chronically inadequate diet (Christian et al., 1998b) and can prevent women from performing their normal household tasks in the evening (Christian et al., 1998a). Keith West described a randomized, community-based trial study conducted in the Terai region of Nepal that examined linkages between vitamin A or beta-carotene supplements and maternal mortality. Giving nonpregnant and pregnant Nepalese women weekly vitamin A or beta-carotene supplements at recommended dietary levels increased vitamin A status by 40 percent and reduced mortality related to pregnancy by 49 percent (West et al., 1999). Vitamin A's role in enhancing resistance to infection provides one plausible explanation for this effect. There may be antioxidant-mediated health effects of beta-carotene, beyond its provitamin A role. Supplementation also reduced the risk of anemia in women who were not infected with hookworm (Dreyfuss, 1998). Although the study results are promising, there were a few incongruous findings, and additional studies are needed in different settings to clarify the mechanism and confirm the role of vitamin A in preventing maternal mortality.

Domestic Violence and Maternal Morbidity

Jacquelyn Campbell discussed recent findings regarding abuse and its relationship to pregnancy, childbirth, and general reproductive health. A recent study in Leon, Nicaragua, found that the lifetime prevalence of spousal violence was 52 percent among ever-married women (Ellsberg et al., 1999). Although there are no global estimates of domestic violence during pregnancy, between 16 and 52 percent of women worldwide are estimated to have ever been physically assaulted by a partner (World Health Organization, 1999). Estimates vary widely due to differences in the survey instruments used to screen women for violence and the sensitive nature of asking such questions.

Physical abuse is not necessarily more prevalent during pregnancy than at other times during a relationship. Some studies indicate a lower prevalence of abuse during pregnancy (Gielen et al., 1994; Gazmararian et al., 1995; Gazmararian et al., 1996). For some women, pregnancy may be a "protected" time in their lives. In other cases, pregnancy may be a cause of anger and violent behavior for abusers, including jealousy of the unborn child or the abuser's attempt to cause a miscarriage. According to Campbell, although the dynamics may change during pregnancy, domestic abuse is usually part of an ongoing pattern.

The mental health effects of abuse during pregnancy are not clear. It is likely that battered pregnant women experience increased depression and anxiety, but there have not been studies of these phenomena. Campbell discussed the possible links between postpartum depression and abuse and between abuse and posttraumatic stress disorder, which has been found in the general population (Campbell, 1998). Abuse during pregnancy has also been linked to low birthweight, even when other risk factors are taken into account (Bullock and McFarlane, 1989; Schei et al., 1991; Parker et al., 1994). This may be due directly to abdominal trauma, infection, or exacerbation of chronic problems (e.g., hypertension or diabetes), or indirectly to stress, or associated with other risk factors, such as substance abuse. Assessments during the antenatal and postpartum period may be the only time that health workers are able to identify abused women and offer services (Campbell, 1998).

Indirect Evidence: Consequences for Children, Families, and Society

There is a significant amount of knowledge about the consequences of frequently repeated pregnancies or acute reproductive and maternal morbidities for women and newborns and their health. However, very little is known about the social and economic consequences of such morbidity for children, families, and ultimately society as a whole. There is little research on the social and economic effects of maternal morbidity particularly, but it is likely to have consequences that are similar to those of other adult illnesses and disabilities, about which some work has been done.

Table 2 shows some of the potential social and economic effects that adult illness may have on the household, both directly and through the implementation of coping processes or efforts to reduce the direct impact. For example, the reduced productivity of an ill adult often results in a reallocation of labor. Medical costs for his or her treatment may require changes in household consumption, saving, and investment patterns. A study presented by Mead Over and Julia Dayton at the workshop showed that morbidity (due to any type of disease or injury, not just reproductive or maternal problems) reduced household consumption. More research is needed to examine the relationship between morbidity and household consumption, but it may be that children living in households with ill mothers are less likely to receive adequate nutrition, and, as noted above, older children may drop out of school to assume some of the mother's responsibilities. Children may also suffer from psychological problems, including feelings of depression and isolation.

OPPORTUNITIES FOR FURTHER RESEARCH

The studies presented at the workshop helped to outline some of the potential linkages between maternal morbidity and maternal mortality and social, economic, and health outcomes for women, their families, and their communities. Although maternal morbidity and mortality may be a large burden in many societies, they are not the only types of illness and injury affecting women or their families. A family's coping mechanisms may be the same whether a woman died in childbirth or due to another cause. Discovering what these coping mechanisms are and especially how they affect children is important for determining effective interventions and further research. Some participants argued that it is important to focus primarily on pregnancy-related morbidity and mortality because it is a significant disease burden for women, and pregnancy is the time when women should be provided with access to the health care system. However, nonpregnant women also often lack adequate access to health care, so access is important for all women, regardless of age or reproductive status, especially if pregnancy delaying, spacing, and limiting measures are being considered.

Much more research is needed before the relationships between maternal morbidity and mortality and the consequences for women, children, families, and society are clearly understood. Generally, however, the evidence indicates that the negative effects are most measurable for individual families and less obvious at the community or societal level. Negative outcomes may be ameliorated by coping mechanisms such as assistance from the extended family or through public welfare programs. Preventing deaths by increasing access to essential obstetric care and also encouraging better nutrition, increased education, improving reproductive health, and expanding access to all types of health care and other services for all women is clearly a desirable objective. The Workshop on the Consequences of Pregnancy, Maternal Morbidity, and Mortality for Women, Their Families, and Society was obviously a starting point for looking at these interrelationships. It is hoped that this report will help to highlight where efforts and resources are most needed.

References

AbouZahr, C., and E. Royston
    1991 *Maternal Mortality: A Global Factbook.* Geneva, Switzerland: World Health Organization.

Ainsworth, M., and I. Semali
    1998 The impact of adult deaths on the nutritional status of children. Ch. 9 in *Coping with AIDS: The Economic Impact of Adult Mortality on the African Household.* Washington, D.C.: World Bank.

Arrowsmith, S., E.C. Hamlin, and L.L. Wall
    1996 Obstructed labor injury complex: Obstetric fistula formation and the multifaceted morbidity of maternal birth trauma in the developing world. *Obstetric and Gynecological Survey* 51(9):568-574.

Basu, A.M.
    1998 The Household Impact of Adult Mortality and Morbidity. Unpublished paper presented at the Workshop on the Consequences of Pregnancy, Maternal Morbidity, and Mortality for Women, Their Families, and Society, Committee on Population, October 19-20, 1998. Available from Division of Nutritional Sciences, Cornell University.

Black, R.E.
    1998 Therapeutic and preventive effects of zinc on serious childhood infectious diseases in developing countries. *American Journal of Clinical Nutrition* 68:476S-479S.

Bullock, L.F., and J. McFarlane
    1989 The birthweight/battering connection. *American Journal of Nursing* 89:1153-1155.

Campbell, J.C.
    1998 Abuse during pregnancy: Progress, policy and potential. *American Journal of Public Health* 88(2):185-187.

Cates, W., Jr.
    1995 Sexually transmitted diseases. Pp. 57-84 in *Reproductive Health Care for Women and Babies,* Benjamin Sachs, Richard Beard, Emile Papiernik, and Cristine Russell, eds. New York: Oxford University Press.

REFERENCES

Chen, L.C., M. Rahman, S. D'Souza, J. Chakraborty, A.M. Sardar, and M.D. Yunus
    1983 Mortality impact of an MCH-FP program in Matlab, Bangladesh. *Studies in Family Planning* 14(8/9):199-209.

Christian, P., A.L. Thorne-Lyman, K.P. West, Jr., M.E. Bentley, S.K. Khatry, E.K. Pradhan, S.C. LeClerq, and S.R. Shrestha
    1998a Working after the sun goes down: Exploring how night blindness impairs women's work activities in rural Nepal. *European Journal of Clinical Nutrition* 52:519-524.

Christian, P., K.P. West, Jr., S.K. Khatry, J. Katz, S.R. Shrestha, E.K. Pradhan, S.C. LeClerq, and R.P. Pokhrel
    1998b Night blindness of pregnancy in rural Nepal—nutritional and health risks. *International Journal of Epidemiology* 27:231-237.

Cobra, C., Muhilal, K. Rusmil, D. Rustama, Djatnika, S.S. Suwardi, D. Permaesih, K. Muherdiyantiningsih, S. Martuti, and R.D. Semba
    1997 Infant survival is improved by oral iodine supplementation. *Journal of Nutrition* 127:574-578.

Cottingham, J., and E. Royston
    1991 *Obstetric Fistulae: A Review of Available Information.* Geneva, Switzerland: World Health Organization.

Dreyfuss, M.L.
    1998 Anemia and Iron Deficiency During Pregnancy: Etiologies and Effects on Birth Outcomes in Nepal. Doctoral dissertation, Johns Hopkins University, Baltimore, MD.

D'Souza, S.
    1994 Death in the Family and Poverty. Unpublished paper presented at seminar on poverty, International Union for the Scientific Study of Population, Florence, 1994. Available from International Population Concerns, Brussels, Belgium.

D'Souza, S., P. Mutijima Nkaka, F. Katangulia, A. Mukiza Gichondo, and F. Nsabimana
    1998 *Socio-Demographic Survey 1996.* Final Report. Ministry of Finance and Economic Planning, National Population Office and United Nations Population Fund, Kigali, Rwanda.

Egypt Ministry of Health
    1994 *National Maternal Mortality Study: Egypt, 1992-1993. Preliminary Report of Findings and Conclusions.* Cairo: Child Survival Project.

Ellsberg, M.C., R. Pena, A. Herrera, J. Liljestrand, and A. Winkvist
    1999 Wife abuse among women of childbearing age in Nicaragua. *American Journal of Public Health* 89(2):241-244.

Gazmararian, J.A., M.M. Adams, L.E. Saltzman, C.H. Johnson, F.C. Bruce, J.S. Marks, and S.C. Zahniser
    1995 The relationship between pregnancy intendedness and physical violence in mothers of newborns. *Obstetrics and Gynecology* 85(6):1031-1038.

Gazmararian, J.A., S. Lazorick, A.M. Spitz, T.J. Ballard, L.E. Saltzman, and J.S. Marks
    1996 Prevalence of violence against pregnant women: A review of the literature. *Journal of the American Medical Association* 275:1915-1920.

Gielen, A.C., P.J. O'Campo, R.R. Faden, N.E. Kass, and X. Xue
    1994 Interpersonal conflict and physical violence during the childbearing year. *Social Science and Medicine* 39:781-787.

Gray, R.H., M.J. Wawer, D. Serwadda, N. Sewankambo, C. Li, F. Wabwire-Mangen, L. Paxton, N. Kiwanuka, G. Kigozi, J. Konde-Lule, T.C. Quinn, C.A. Gaydos, and D. McNairn
    1998 Population-based study of fertility in women with HIV-1 infection in Uganda. *Lancet* 351:98-103.

REFERENCES

Harrison, K.A., U.G. Lister, C.E. Rossiter, and H. Chong
   1985   Child-bearing, health and social priorities: A survey of 22,774 consecutive hospital births in Zaria, Northern Nigeria. *British Journal of Obstetrics and Gynecology* 92:86-99.

Katz, J., S.K. Khatry, K.P. West, Jr., J.H. Humphrey, S.C. LeClerq, E.K. Pradhan, R.P. Pokhrel, and A. Sommer
   1995   Night blindness is prevalent during pregnancy and lactation in rural Nepal. *Journal of Nutrition* 125:2122-2127.

Llewellyn-Jones, D.
   1965   Severe anemia in pregnancy. *Australia and New Zealand Journal of Obstetrics and Gynecology* 5:191-197.

Merialdi, M., L.E. Caulfield, N. Zavaleta, A. Figueroa, and J.A. DiPietro
   1999   Adding zinc to prenatal iron and folate tablets improves fetal neurobehavioral development. *American Journal of Obstetrics and Gynecology* 180:483-490.

Murphy, J.F., J. O'Riordan, R.G. Newcombe, E.C. Coles, and J.F. Peason
   1986   Relation of hemoglobin levels in first and second trimesters to outcome of pregnancy. *Lancet* 1(8488):992-994.

National Research Council
   1989   *Contraception and Reproduction: Health Consequences for Women and Children in the Developing World.* Working Group on the Health Consequences of Contraceptive Use and Controlled Fertility, Committee on Population, Commission on Behavioral and Social Sciences and Education, National Research Council. Washington, D.C.: National Academy Press.

Parker, B., J. McFarlane, and K. Soeken
   1994   Abuse during pregnancy: Effects on maternal complications and birth weight in adult and teenage women. *American Journal of Obstetrics and Gynecology* 84:323-328.

Preziosi, P., A. Prual, P. Galan, H. Daouda, H. Boureima, and S. Hercberg
   1997   Effect of iron supplementation on the iron status of pregnant women: Consequences for newborns. *American Journal of Clinical Nutrition* 66:1178-1182.

Schei, B., S.O. Samuelsen, and L.S. Bakketeig
   1991   Does spousal physical abuse affect the outcome of pregnancy? *Scandinavian Journal of Social Medicine* 19:26-31.

Strong, M.A.
   1998   The Effects of Adult Mortality on Infant and Child Mortality. Unpublished paper presented at the Workshop on the Consequences of Pregnancy, Maternal Morbidity and Mortality for Women, Their Families, and Society, Committee on Population, October 19-20, 1998. Available from U.S. Agency for International Development, Nairobi, Kenya.

United Nations
   1999   *World Population Prospects, The 1998 Revision, Vol. I, Comprehensive Tables.* New York: United Nations.

West, K.P., Jr., J. Katz, S.K. Khatry, S.C. LeClerq, E.K. Pradhan, S.R. Shrestha, P.B. Connor, S.M. Dali, P.Christian, R.P. Pokhrel, A. Sommer, and the NNIPS-2 Study Group
   1999   Double blind, cluster randomised trial of low dose supplementation with vitamin A or beta carotene on mortality related to pregnancy in Nepal. *British Medical Journal* 318:570-575.

World Bank
   1993   *World Development Report 1993: Investing in Health.* New York: Oxford University Press.
   1997   *Confronting AIDS: Public Priorities in a Global Epidemic.* New York: Oxford University Press.

World Health Organization
- 1992 *International Classification of Diseases and Related Health Problems, Tenth Revision.* Vol. 1. Geneva, Switzerland: World Health Organization.
- 1993 *Making Maternity Care More Accessible.* Press Release No. 59. Geneva, Switzerland: World Health Organization.
- 1994 *Mother-Baby Package: Implementing safe motherhood in countries.* Publication number WHO/FHE/MSM/94.11. Geneva, Switzerland: World Health Organization.
- 1997 *Maternal Health Around the World.* Wall chart available from Department of Reproductive Health and Research, World Health Organization, Geneva, Switzerland.
- 1999 Violence Against Women Information Pack: A Priority Health Issue. Available electronically: *http://www.who.int/frhwhd/VAW/infopack/English/VAW.infopack.htm#* [March 2, 1999].

World Health Organization and United Nations Children's Fund
- 1996 *Revised 1990 Estimates of Maternal Mortality: A New Approach by WHO and UNICEF.* Geneva, Switzerland: World Health Organization.

Yip, R.
- 1994 Iron deficiency: Contemporary scientific issues and international programmatic approaches. *Journal of Nutrition* 124:1479S-1490S.

Zhou, L.M., W.W. Yang, J.Z. Hua, C.Q. Deng, X. Tao, and R.J. Stoltzfus
- 1998 Relation of hemoglobin measured at different times in pregnancy to preterm birth and low birth weight in Shanghai, China. *American Journal of Epidemiology* 148:998-1006.

APPENDIX A

Definitions

REPRODUCTIVE MORBIDITY

The World Health Organization (1992) has defined reproductive morbidity as consisting of three types of morbidity: obstetric, gynecologic, and contraceptive. (Obstetric morbidity is the equivalent of maternal morbidity.)

Obstetric morbidity—morbidity in a woman who has been pregnant (regardless of the site or duration of the pregnancy) from any cause related to or aggravated by the pregnancy or its management, but not from accidental or incidental causes.

1. *Direct obstetric morbidity* results from obstetric complications of the pregnant state (pregnancy, labor, and the puerperium), from interventions, omissions, incorrect treatment, or from a chain of events resulting from any of the above. This can include temporary conditions, mild or severe, which occur during pregnancy or within 42 days of delivery, or permanent/chronic conditions resulting from pregnancy, abortion or childbirth. Some chronic conditions (such as anemia or hypertension) may be caused by pregnancy and delivery, but are equally likely to have other causes.

2. *Indirect obstetric morbidity* results from a previously existing condition or disease, such as sickle cell disease or tuberculosis, which was aggravated by the physiologic effects of pregnancy. Such morbidity may occur at any time and continue beyond the reproductive years.

3. *Psychological obstetric morbidity* may include puerperal psychosis, at-

tempted suicide, strong fear of pregnancy and childbirth, and may be the consequence of obstetric complications, obstetric interventions, cultural practices (such as isolation during labor and delivery), or coercion.

Gynecologic morbidity—includes any condition, disease, or dysfunction of the reproductive system which is not related to pregnancy, abortion, or childbirth, but may be related to sexual behavior.

1. *Direct gynecologic morbidity* includes reproductive cancers, premenstrual syndrome (PMS), endocrine system disorders, bacterial or viral sexually transmitted diseases (STDs) and their sequelae (cervical cancer, pelvic inflammatory disease [PID], secondary sterility, AIDS), reproductive tract infections (RTIs), coital injuries.
2. *Indirect gynecologic morbidity* includes primarily traditional practices, some of which are for treatment of real or perceived gynecologic conditions (such as female genital mutilation, gishiri cuts).
3. *Psychological morbidity* includes psychological disorders associated with STDs, infertility, traditional practices, dyspareunia, fistulae, rape.

Contraceptive morbidity—includes conditions which result from efforts (other than abortion) to limit fertility, whether they are traditional or modern methods. Examples include menorrhagia from IUD use, thromboses from oral contraceptive use, and wound infections after Norplant insertion.

MATERNAL MORTALITY

Maternal morbidity (or obstetric morbidity as defined above) can lead in turn to death. Death due to pregnancy-related causes is known as maternal mortality or maternal death. Maternal death is officially defined by the World Health Organization (1992:1238):

> [T]he death of a woman while pregnant or within 42 days of termination of pregnancy, irrespective of the duration and the site of the pregnancy, from any cause related to or aggravated by the pregnancy or its management, but not from accidental or incidental causes.

WHO subdivides maternal deaths into two groups:

1. *Direct obstetric deaths* are those deaths resulting from obstetric complications of the pregnant state (pregnancy, labor, and puerperium), from interventions, omissions, incorrect treatment, or from a chain of events resulting from any of the above.

2. *Indirect obstetric deaths* are those resulting from previous existing disease or disease that developed during pregnancy and which was not due to direct obstetric causes, but which was aggravated by physiologic effects of pregnancy.

WHO defines two other specific types of maternal mortality. A *late maternal death* is the death of a woman from direct or indirect obstetric causes more than 42 days but less than 1 year after termination of pregnancy. A *pregnancy-related death* is the death of a woman while pregnant or within 42 days of termination of pregnancy, irrespective of the cause of death.

APPENDIX B

Workshop Agenda

Workshop on the Consequences of Pregnancy, Maternal Morbidity, and Mortality for Women, Their Families, and Society

October 19-20, 1998

Committee on Population
National Research Council of the National Academy of Sciences
2101 Constitution Avenue, NW
NAS Board Room
Washington, DC

October 19

CONSEQUENCES OF MATERNAL MORBIDITY

8:30 Continental Breakfast

9:15 Welcome
      Faith Mitchell, National Research Council

9:30 Introduction
      Marjorie Koblinsky, MotherCare/John Snow, Inc.
      Joy Riggs-Perla, U.S. Agency for International Development

Consequences of Pregnancy Complications and Problems Associated with Pregnancy

9:45 Obstructed Labor and Its Consequences
      Lewis Wall, Louisiana State University Medical Center and
      Tulane University School of Public Health and Tropical Medicine

10:15 Comments
      Jason Smith, Family Health International

10:30	Discussion
10:45	Break

11:00	Association Between HIV/AIDS and Reduced Fertility in Rakai, Uganda, and in the United States
	   Ronald Gray, Johns Hopkins University
	   Lisa M. Lee, Centers for Disease Control and Prevention

11:45	Effects of STIs on Women's Fertility and Pregnancy Outcomes Ward Cates, Family Health International
12:15	Comments Jane Menken, University of Colorado at Boulder
12:30	Discussion
1:00	Lunch

Maternal Nutrition

2:00	Maternal Nutritional Depletion from Frequent Reproductive Cycling: Revisiting the Issues Ten Years Later Kathleen Merchant, University of Nevada, Las Vegas
2:30	The Effects of Maternal Vitamin A and Beta-Carotene Supplementation on Birth Outcomes in Nepal: A Randomized Community Trial Keith West, Johns Hopkins University
3:00	Comments Reynaldo Martorell, Emory University
3:15	Discussion
3:30	Break

ADVERSE CONSEQUENCES ON PREGNANCY

3:45	Abuse During Pregnancy as a Risk Factor on Morbidity and Other Consequences Jacquelyn Campbell, Johns Hopkins University

4:15	Association Between High Parity/Short Birth Spacing and Child and Maternal Mortality Carine Ronsmans, London School of Hygiene and Tropical Medicine
4:45	Comments Shea Rutstein, MEASURE/DHS+
5:00	Discussion
5:30	Adjourn
6:00	Reception
7:00	Dinner

October 20

CONSEQUENCES OF MATERNAL MORTALITY

8:30	Continental Breakfast
9:15	Introduction to the Consequences of Maternal Mortality Henry Mosley, Johns Hopkins University

Consequences of Maternal Mortality for Children

9:30	Consequences of Parental Death for Child Survival in Bangladesh Michael Strong, U.S. Agency for International Development
10:00	Consequences of the Death of a Mother or Other Female Household Member on Children's Schooling and Nutrition in Tanzania Martha Ainsworth, The World Bank
10:30	Break
10:45	Comments Sonalde Desai, University of Maryland
11:00	Discussion

Socioeconomic Consequences of Maternal Mortality for the Family and Society

11:30	The Impact of Maternal Morbidity and Mortality on Household Consumption in Kagera, Tanzania
	    Mead Over, The World Bank
	    Julia Dayton, Yale University (co-author)
	    Phare Mujinja, University of Dar es Salaam (co-author)

12:00	Social and Other Consequences of Parental Death: Examples from Kinshasa and Kigali Stan D'Souza, International Population Concerns
12:30	Discussion
1:00	Lunch
2:00	Potential Household Impact of Adult Mortality in India Alaka Basu, Cornell University
2:15	Comments Anne Tinker, The World Bank
2:30	Discussion

3:00	Discussion of Possible Next Steps
	    Marjorie Koblinsky, MotherCare/John Snow, Inc.
	    Henry Mosley, Johns Hopkins University

3:30	Discussion
4:30	Adjourn